Thinking of...

Joining a gym?

Ask the Smart Questions

By Frank Bennett

_____

Disclaimer

The purpose of this book is to help you make a decision about joining a gym and create the foundations for an active and healthy lifestyle. Neither the author nor publisher is offering medical advice other than to report on that which is in the public domain.

Always consult your doctor to discuss any concerns that you may have before commencing an exercise programme.

Smart Questions™ Philosophy

Smart Questions is built on 4 key pillars, which set it apart from other publishers:

1. *Smart people want Smart Questions not Dumb Answers*
2. *Domain experts are often excluded from authorship, so we are making writing a book simple and painless*
3. *The community has a great deal to contribute to enhance the content*
4. *We donate a percentage of revenue to a charity voted for by the authors and community. It is great marketing, but it is also the right thing to do*

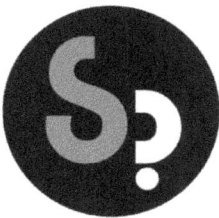

www.Smart-Questions.com

5 a day

Eat more fruit and vegetables, 5 portions a day is recommended

5 a week

Exercise for 30 minutes a day on 5 or more days a week

1 life, your life

You make the choices

Author

Frank Bennett

Frank is a REPs Level 4 Advanced Instructor[1] and a member of the Fitness Industry Association. He has numerous qualifications to instruct various exercise classes and work with special needs clients to include those referred by their doctor for exercise and those diagnosed as obese. He has experience in gyms in the public sector, corporate sector and private member clubs and currently manages a team of fitness instructors and personal trainers at a leisure centre.

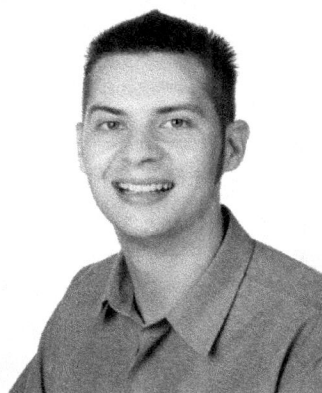

www.thinkingofjoiningagym.co.uk

---

[1] The Register of Exercise Professionals (REPs) web site at
http://www.exerciseregister.org/ has a list of all REPs qualified fitness instructors.

Table of Contents

1 Your health, it's personal 1

2 They think they know best 7

3 You know what's best 11

4 GROW and be well 15

5 Ask the Smart Questions 17

6 This probably can't wait Questions 21

7 Questions for me 23

8 Questions for them.. 31

9 Other People.. 39

10 A secret revealed 45

11 Final Word 49

Acknowledgements

In some way every client that I have worked with has in some part contributed to my writing this book. It has been fascinating to meet people with aspirations to make a change in their life to improve their health and wellbeing and see how that transformation unfolds over time – more on this later.

This book is a consumer's guide and has been topic of many conversations with people that have joined gyms and left, current gym members and those that have never considered joining a gym. Their input provided the reality check.

In writing this book, I have involved my father who has contributed from his experience as a gym member and from running membership sales teams for gym operators.

I want to thank a number of people who have taken an interest and contributed to the writing of this book:

The team at the Fitness Industry Association (you know who you are) for their guidance.

John Wileman, President of the Institute of Sports and Recreation Management for his review of the book.

Marcia Hammond a Podiatrist (foot specialist) registered with the Society of Chiropodists and Podiatrists for her advice on choosing footwear for exercise and health care advice for feet.

Preface

Joining a gym represents a commitment to your health and wellbeing that entails the allocation your time and money albeit for a good purpose. You will want to be sure that it is the right decision for you. A search online using Google or your favourite search engine overwhelms you with information whereas this book is compact in providing insight and information to help you ask the smart questions so you make the right decision for you.

It is the case that our health, wellbeing and appearance is being elevated as something of importance: Fat Club, Celebrity Fit Club, 10 Years Younger, My Big Fat Diet Show, How to Look Good Naked are just a few of the many TV programmes that look at how people cope with their anxieties.

Do you worry about your weight or your appearance? Who does not at heart want to look good and feel-good? This in not illusive – it is about choices – and a commitment to change some things in your life such as healthy eating and regular exercise.

Some things in life are under our control and some are not but there is no doubt that your health, barring accident or misfortune, is something that you control. When people say, you look 'fit and healthy', that is a statement of admiration and much as you will appreciate the compliment; how you feel about yourself is what really matters.

This is as personal as it gets – your health, your wellbeing.

Who should read this book?

This book is intended as a catalyst for action. Here are a few examples of people and life's situations that might be applicable?

Health scare? Perhaps you have been to your doctor and they have informed you that you have high blood pressure and advised you start up an exercise programme. They may have also prescribed medication.

Relationship problems? Many people make a personal commitment to their health and fitness following the breakup of a relationship.

Big event ahead? Perhaps you are getting married or going on the holiday of a lifetime and want to look your best.

Gagging for a compliment? Not many of those around today are there. Perhaps you feel the tonic is in getting fit rather than in a gin and tonic?

Sex life evaporated? Surveys reveal it reported commonplace that general health, body image and energy levels all affect a sex life.

Sporting event ahead? Perhaps you have entered a marathon or half marathon or a charity bike ride? You need to prepare and do so in a way that you avoid injury.

Clothes shrunk? On the other hand, did you just get bigger? Looked at the price of a new wardrobe and had the thought; there has to be a better way?

Something hit a nerve? There are plenty of reports about personal health matters in newspapers, magazines, on TV and online. Did something hit home?

Had this moment? Don't take this wrong way but...

Happy as you are or are you ready for change?

A special message for families

Later in this book I talk about the growing problem of obesity and its health consequences. The news is not good as research shows that obesity among both males and females is growing with the sharpest rise reported among those aged 18-30 when physically you are in the prime of your life. Many people in this age group will be parents and so I wanted to send a special message to you.

No matter your age if you are a parent or guardian then consider that the attitudes that you have toward your health has a direct influence on your children. For example, if you exercise it is likely that you will encourage your children to exercise and if you choose to eat healthy foods (with the occasional indulgence – we are only human) then your children will eat similarly.

The UK government has invested in Change4Life to provide encouragement and support for families to lead a healthy lifestyle that incorporates good eating habits and exercise. This campaign has many supporters including supermarkets and gyms and it is easy to join in. Go to *www.nhs.uk/change4life*

If you are thinking of joining a gym, why not make it a family activity?

If you have special needs

This book does not assume that you are able-bodied while it does presume you are capable of self-action. I myself work with clients with medical conditions referred to me by their doctor and others that are living with disability.

If your doctor refers you for exercise (exercise referral) they will know which gyms have specialist trained staff to support you.

If you have a disability then you will be interested in the Inclusive Fitness Initiative (IFI) details at *http://www.inclusivefitness.org*. Here you will find information about gyms that cater for the needs of disabled persons. The web site also provides a postcode lookup to find gyms in your local area that have IFI accredited facilities.

How to use this book

This book is intended as a catalyst for action. I hope that the ideas and examples inspire you to act. So, do whatever you need to do to make this book useful. Many people opt to involve a friend so go to our website and email them the e-book summary.

This symbol is used throughout the book to draw your attention to an idea or something to consider – I hope that helps.

Chapter

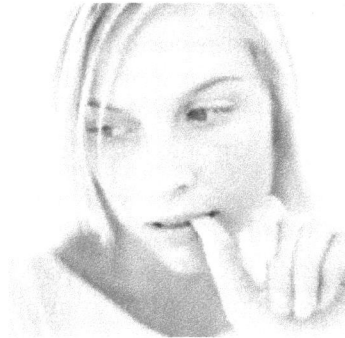

Your health, it's personal

It's choice – not chance – that determines your destiny.

Jean Nidetch (founder of the Weight Watchers organization, 1923 –)

WORKING out, getting fit, leading an active lifestyle requires effort. Why make the effort when you can have most things done by paying someone else to do it?

Your house is in a mess because you have not made the effort to clean and tidy. No problem, pay someone to clean it up. We pay to alleviate the effort of many things in life. Your health is not something you can delegate or pay someone else, you get to look after it – it is a special relationship.

Do not be lulled into thinking that your doctor looks after your health. That is your responsibility. Your doctor will help you get well again when you are sick. If your doctor diagnoses your health problem being connected with your lifestyle they may talk to you about making changes, such as taking more exercise or modifying your diet (what you eat and how much you eat).

It is popular to see people featured on TV programmes resorting to cosmetic surgery to repair and rejuvenate their body and presumably their image. This is an option but surgery comes with risks, is expensive and beyond the financial reach of most people. Besides, when did you last hear someone say; I had surgery last week it was a lot of fun and I cannot wait to have some more.

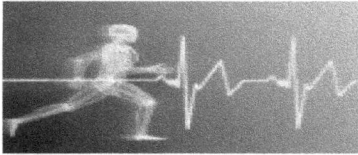

It's your body - it is your most precious thing - unique - yours - you own it and get to look after it or neglect it - you make the choice.

It is your choice and in a world flooded with 'look good feel-good' advertisements and glossy images of the good life we are urged to lead, one thing remains true; the power of choice is yours alone. This is exactly what Jean Nidetch was referring to; if you don't like the way things are then change it – you have the power of choice.

In a world that is, whether you like it or not, increasingly aware of the health risks associated with lifestyle choices we all need to find a balance between enjoying life and at the same time keeping well.

The paradox is that if we enjoy life too much through over-indulgence in foods or alcohol then our health can suffer and that impairs the enjoyment of life. The current statistics on obesity[2] are evidence that many people have the wrong balance and face potentially chronic health problems.

Looking around you will have noticed we all have the same body parts it is just that we make different choices about how we look after the body. This is in part biological and in other part the choices we make. For example as you read the table opposite do the comments in one column better represent the choices you make in your life?

---

[2] Obesity is when a person is carrying too much body fat for their height and sex. A person is considered obese if they have a Body Mass Index (BMI) of 30 or greater. Source: NHS *www.nhs.uk*. BMI is explained in Chapter 2.

I...	I...
Do exercise	Don't or prefer not to exercise
Do not smoke	Smoke
Drink moderately aware of the recommended number of alcohol units per week	I drink pints not units – recommended number – I'll decide
Eat Breakfast	Skip breakfast
Will walk or cycle	Jump in the car - it's quicker
Take the stairs	Take the lift – it's effortless
Say No to snacks – Yes to fruit	Say Yes to snacks - yummy
Avoid Sugar	2, no, make that 3 spoons
Eat only what I need to satisfy my hunger	Fill up until I'm completely stuffed

Life offers plenty of choices and it is not as if the choices are always binary; as in good for you or bad for you - rather that we need to understand the consequences of our choices.

This is not a book about morals, rather it is about the power of choice and the decisions you face for your health and wellbeing.

If you had a blank piece of paper and wrote down how you would like to describe yourself which of the following would you prefer to be about you.

Describing me...	Describing me ...
I'm looking after myself because I want to enjoy good health	I've felt better I know that much but I can't truly remember what that felt like
I feel fit and well and have energy to …	I used to exercise more and now I just don't feel like exercising
I generally sleep well and wake up refreshed	My clothes feel tighter and I'm not so sure anymore what size I take
I know how to control my weight	Stressed
I understand my relationship with chocolate	At the end of a day my feet hurt and I often feel very tired
On a warm and sunny day if someone suggests a bike ride to the beach for a swim my response is – I'm up for that let's go	A bike ride sounds like a nice idea but …
	I don't know my daily calorie intake – why, is that important?
I feel-good about my appearance	I'm not comfortable talking about my appearance

Your body is yours and only you can look after it.

So, you are Thinking of...Joining a gym?

You are exercising the power of choice, so let's help you know if this is the right choice for you by asking the smart questions.

While this book has the title Thinking of…Joining a gym? its core message is about **your health and wellbeing**. The fact is exercise is good for your health and wellbeing. But you get to decide and in demonstration of that the Wordle[3] below takes all the words in this opening chapter and creates a graphic of the words that are most frequently used and expresses that by the size of the words.

Two words stand out, **health** and **choice**.

---

[3] Wordle is a toy for generating "word clouds" from text. The clouds give greater prominence to words that appear more frequently in the source text. *www.wordle.net*

Your health, it's personal

Chapter

2

They think they know best

Everybody gets so much information all day long that they lose their common sense.

Gertrude Stein (US author in France, 1874 – 1946)

PLEASE stop telling me what is good for me, I get a lot of information about how to conduct my life; do this but not that. Let me make up my own mind.

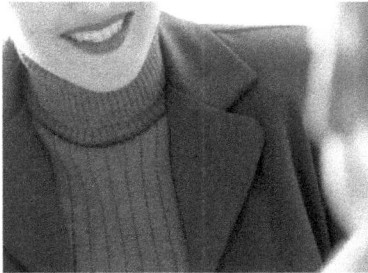

In the chapter 1, we talked about lifestyle choices and since this book is about helping you decide if joining a gym is the right decision for you, we now look at this in more detail. Of course, we don't know what we don't know and that is a reason to read this book.

Many people have made this New Year resolution: I'm going to join a gym and lose weight. Off they go to the gym and they ask you want you want to achieve and you say: "I want to lose weight and tone up." Do you know how many times a fitness instructor will have heard this? I think you can guess.

Evidently many people think that joining a gym is a way to lose weight and tone up? It is one way and for many people it helps them meet their 'lose weight and tone up' objectives. For others they dread the idea and feel intimidated by the unfamiliar setting of a gym.

Next time you are out in a shopping mall or high street look around and make some casual observations about the people you see. What attracts you to some people but not to others? Is it the way they dress? Do they look good in their clothes? Are you struck by their physical appearance; they look fit or need to lose weight. Do they radiate good health? If they do, what emotion does that invoke?

Here is the brunt of the problem; it is easier to be critical of someone else than to make a candid assessment of ourself. Would you agree?

Few people are brave enough to invite someone to offer a candid assessment of their appearance and we all know the little promises that we make to our self only to put them aside until another day. Occasionally something will happen in our life to knock our inertia aside and make something happen.

So, for those who think they know best here is their recipe of advice for you to follow; if you want to?

The Chief Medical Officer's recommendation for health-related activity in adults is:

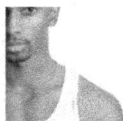

Adults should achieve a total of at least 30 minutes of moderate[4] intensity physical activity a day, on 5 or more days a week

Remove from your mind 30 minutes and substitute the idea that 5 times a week you are going to do something that will you will enjoy and have beneficial effects for your health.

In many ways our life has routine; we brush our teeth at least twice a day, we eat 3 times a day (sometimes more!), we work, we sleep, we relax and we should exercise. Too many times, I hear people talk of exercise as a test of physical ability that they believe results in aches and pains. The reality is coping with illness and disease that are consequence of a lifestyle that does not incorporate exercise is more likely to result in aches and pains and worse.

Look at the next table. Which of these tips do you already follow and which do you think you would have most difficulty to follow?

---

[4] Examples of moderate activity would be walking at 3 mph or cycling at 10-12 mph on a flat road surface.

When you read the tips you may consider them common sense but like many common sense things, actually doing it is something else.

The Chief Medical Officer's Ten Tips For Better Health:

1.	Don't smoke and don't breathe others' tobacco smoke.
2.	Eat at least 5 portions of fruit and vegetables each day and cut down on fat, salt and added sugar.
3.	Be physically active for at least 30 minutes, 5 days a week
4.	Maintain, or aim for, a healthy weight (BMI[5] 20-25).
5.	If you drink alcohol, have no more than 2-3 units[6] a day (women) or 3-4 units a day (men).
6.	Protect yourself from the sun: cover up, keep in the shade, never burn and use factor 15 plus sunscreen. Take extra care to protect children.
7.	Practise safer sex – use a condom.
8.	Make the decision to go for cancer screening when invited.
9.	On the roads, THINK safety.
10.	Manage stress levels - talking things through, relaxation and physical activity can help.

Are any of these tips already in your consciousness?

How did you spontaneously respond when reading the tips? Knew that, do that, should do that but don't, Oops, makes sense, keep meaning to.

Health is a lifestyle choice and something that you might want to think about as a condition of your life.

[5] Body Mass Index (BMI) can be calculated by weight (kg) divided by height (m) squared (i.e.kg/m2). If you weigh 100 kilograms and your height is 2 metres your BMI is 25 (100/4).
[6] A pint of beer is approx. 2 units and a glass of wine is 1.5 – 3 units depending on its size and strength.

The two top reasons why I see people in my gym are to lose weight and to get fit. Here are some options for you to consider:

You want to...	Then do this...
Lose Weight	Go to your doctor or health advisor
Lose Weight	Join Weight Watchers
Lose Weight	Pick out a diet (there are hundreds) from a magazine or online
Get Fit	Buy a Wii-Fit Plus and work out at home
Get Fit	Start walking/running/cycling
Get Fit	Go swimming
Get Fit	Go to the gym

You have lots of choices and for most people a combination of nutritional advice so you eat healthily with an exercise programme that you enjoy and is safe results in weight loss and an improvement in health and fitness. It is as simple as that.

Now where do you go to get qualified advice about combining nutrition and exercise with the facilities to get you started and the support system you will need to help you through your transformation?

Perhaps that is a gym and what you want to know before you commit yourself; is joining a gym the smart choice for me?

Chapter

3

You know what's best

The first step to getting the things you want out of life is this: Decide what you want.

Ben Stein (Author, 1944 –)

ONLY you can decide what is best for you. You can be offered advice, guidance, support, reassurance and incentives but at the end of the day, you will make up your own mind.

Have you considered what is core to your life? Would that include: family, friends, your home life, your career, your personal hopes and ambitions? Do you consider your health core to your life? In general, we do not, because when we are in good health we take it for granted (it is how things are meant to be) and it is only when we get sick that we recognise how much we depend on our health to function in life.

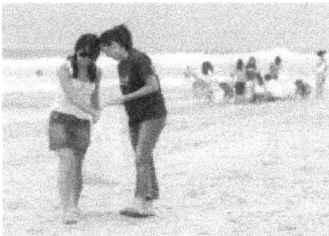

You know the difference it makes when your health is poor as against when you are on form. Can you try to imagine your health improved? It is not easy but the parallel is there and to give an example; think about how much better you feel and look having spent a weekend outdoors perhaps on the beach, you notice it and so do others.

Of course, the underlying challenge is that with today's busy lifestyles and with so many things to do; where do you find the time to indulge you.

So to the point of this chapter; you know what is best for you and you get to decide.

Other than time the next challenge for most people is to elevate in their consciousness the importance of their health and then to think about that as a personal responsibility.

If only we had an Owner's Manual given to us when we were born. What would your Owner's Manual say?

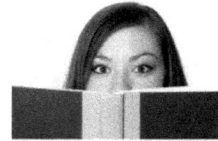

In all likelihood, it would be in many parts:
Looking after you as a child, an adolescent, a young adult, in middle age and as a senior.

In our early life as child and adolescent, we are taken care of by parents and schools so that is delegated and we trust that they know what is best for us. In the case of school, they have trained professionals and guidelines to follow. In the case of parents or guardians that may not be the case as their own lifestyle choices would be a commanding influence, e.g. a sedentary life with little or no exercise vs. an active lifestyle.

You start to exercise your choices as a young adult although to a greater or lesser extent your peers will influence you. These are influential years as you configure your preferred lifestyle that may or may not include sport and recreation. You may have been a talented sportsperson at school or college within an organised activity, but when you leave, you can only continue if you take responsibility for organising your on-going participation perhaps by joining a gym. Often at this stage of life money is short so that makes for difficult choices. All council operated leisure centres offer pay as you go admittance and concessions and you should enquire what is available and check if you qualify.

In middle age, you may have family commitments and/or powering your career ahead and feel overstretched (and stressed) – reported as the time-poor generation. At this time, your health may not be your highest priority yet your busy life depends on you remaining healthy as you have many commitments.

In your senior years, your parenting responsibility may shift from children to looking after parents. Your working life is still busy but the sun is setting on your career and you may have found a comfortable work – life balance. You may have some health problems or know someone who has and are very aware of your physical limitations. You may be wondering what is ahead and how you remain fit and healthy.

These are just typical patterns of life and you may recognise some aspects depending on your age.

Many people associate exercise with physical exertion and disassociate exercise with relaxation. It is a paradox since many people find exercise a way to relax and the beneficial effect of exercise helps relaxation; in the sense of a feeling of wellbeing.

We often seek relaxation when we are stressed but if we are tired, the cure is sleep. Have you tried to relax or sleep when you are stressed? Those that exercise confirm that exercise is great way to alleviate stress so that when you do relax that is quality time and you sleep better.

> Don't think in terms of exercise being at the expense of your time for relaxation as this will almost certainly present you with a dilemma.

Do think in terms of exercise as an element of the time that you set aside for relaxation. You do set aside time for relaxation?

You know what's best

Chapter

4

GROW and be well

Goals allow you to control the direction of change in your favour.

Brian Tracy (Author and Motivational Speaker, 1944 -)

I N our busy lives it is sometimes easy to overlook things that matter, like our health and well being, yet are really important to us. When we are able to put this is context, things become clearer.

The big picture is life, your expectations and hopes for your life, and that can be complex to describe.

A technique used by coaches to help you work through this is referred to as GROW.

G for your Goals – how do you choose to describe these?

R for your Reality – what is reality for you?

O for your Options – what are your viable options?

W for your Will – what will you commit to to achieve your goals?

Use the table opposite to describe your GROW comparing side-by-side two aspects of your life.

	Your work/ family / study etc.	Your health and wellbeing
Goals – my goals are		
Reality – my reality is		
Options – my options are		
Will – I will commit to...		

This simple exercise will highlight your attitudes toward your health and wellbeing. There is no right or wrong in setting your goals, after all they are personal to you.

Which of the two columns did you find easier to complete?

What does that inform you to do now?

Did you recognise you need to give more priority to your health and wellbeing?

Chapter

5

Ask the Smart Questions

If I have seen further it is by standing on the shoulders of giants

Isaac Newton (Scientist, 1643 – 1727)

S
O it is time to start thinking about your choices and what you consider to be in your best interests. To do that you need to confront some things beforehand, such as your future.

The choices you make today can't change what has already happened in your life but they surely do affect your future and much of the public health advice that you receive today is about your future health.

Here is the deal on offer. When you increase physical activity so it becomes habit (5 times a week) then your health and sense of wellbeing benefits with a decrease in body fat and body weight, increase in bone density, lower blood pressure, improved lung function, improved mood, reduced stress and anxiety, increased energy levels and improved mobility. Sound good?

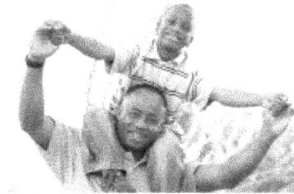

Think these things might apply to you but are not sure then go to the Fitness Industry Association web site and take their health survey at:

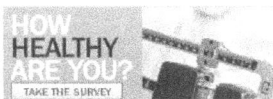

http://www.fia.org.uk/health-and-activity.html

A big public health concern for people of all ages is obesity. You are not born obese it is something that develops over time and the major worry is that it is now evident in young children.

All the studies show that obesity is on the increase and the health consequences are serious to include: heart disease, diabetes, kidney failure, osteoarthritis, back pain and psychological damage[7].

As a recent government report highlights: on present trends obesity will soon surpass smoking as the greatest cause of premature loss of life (in other words death). Most people are aware as a result of government campaigning and advertising that smoking can cause death through lung cancer. To hear the news that being obese can be a cause of death will be a surprise to many and alarming to those that are obese. This is big (no pun intended) and important news.

The report remarks: it is important to recognise that obesity is both a medical condition and a lifestyle disorder and both factors have to be seen within a context of individual, family and societal functioning.

I think most people will understand what a medical condition, but a lifestyle disorder.

My research reveals there is no single definition for lifestyle disorder but in practical terms, it is all about the choices we make, or in your case, you make.

To keep it simple, if you want to avoid the complications of medical conditions that are consequence of your lifestyle choices then you need to balance what you eat and how much you eat with the amount of exercise you take. Since you eat every day, you have to think about exercising everyday as well. This is a lifestyle choice – your choice. It is a lifestyle disorder when you make the wrong choices – you eat too much and do not exercise.

We already know the recommendation that an adult exercise at least 30 minutes of moderate intensity physical activity a day, on 5 or more days a week.

So how much should we eat? That depends on many factors. For example if you work in an office and spend many hours desk bound then your needs are quite different to a manual labourer.

---

[7] As reported in the House of Commons Health Committee Report on Obesity printed 10 May 2004.

Your age and sex also need taken into account. The NHS has an excellent web site with advice and a healthy eating self-assessment tool. See Appendix for how to access these resources.

Gyms are an industry and exist for a reason; to provide you a place where expert advice is available so you can enjoy exercise in a safe environment and have fun!

All gyms employ trained professionals to provide you with the help, advice and support that you need and for most people is a better way than a 'go it alone' approach and you will make friends with others and experience the camaraderie of a gym.

There are more than 6000 gyms in the UK offering a range of facilities and they cater for all ages, interests and abilities. Most gyms are open 7 days a week typically between the hours of 6.00 a.m. and 10.00 p.m. Availability is not a limiting factor with 90% of the population living within 2 miles of a gym or leisure centre[8].

Not sure where to look for help and information about gyms in your area then go to the Fitness Industry Association web site at

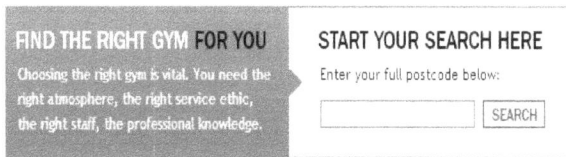

FIND THE RIGHT GYM FOR YOU   **START YOUR SEARCH HERE**

Choosing the right gym is vital. You need the right atmosphere, the right service ethic, the right staff, the professional knowledge.

Enter your full postcode below:

[   ] SEARCH

http://www.fia.org.uk/find-a-gym.html put in your postcode and a list will be provided.

When it comes to your health that is personal and however much information you have available to you only you know the importance of your health?

In the following chapters we look at helping you evaluate this question.

---

[8] Source: Fitness Industry Association at www.fia.org.uk

Ask the Smart Questions

Chapter

6

This probably can't wait Questions

One's first step in wisdom is to question everything - and one's last is to come to terms with everything.

Georg Christoph Lichtenberg (Scientist, 1742 – 1799)

ONE of the biggest challenges for so many is configuring the day to balance all your commitments and some days it just seems you run out of time to do all the things you said you would do.

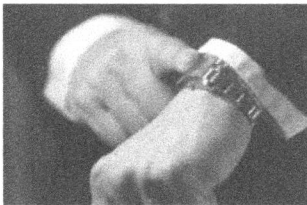

Went to work early intending to finish early but finished late. Started something and it took much longer than you ever imagined. Something came up that couldn't wait and that was your day. It happens.

There is no secret to managing your time but you can do some things to prepare for the unexpected. Be prepared for the time that does become available to exercise and here are some practical tips: always have available a pair of walking boots, your gym kit and swimming gear with a fresh towel and leave it in the car or at the office, whatever works for you. Then when the opportunity arises you are ready to go. Easy.

As you are thinking of joining a gym, I have arranged the following two chapters with questions 'for me' and questions 'for them' the gyms that you visit. Remember to take the book with you to remind you of what is important to you.

This probably can't wait Questions

Chapter

7

Questions for me

Our lives improve only when we take chances - and the first and most difficult risk we can take is to be honest with ourselves.

Walter Anderson (Writer, 1885 - 1962)

DO you think you take fewer chances in life by taking no action or by taking action? When you look back at life most things likely happened because you took positive action. Is that true for you?

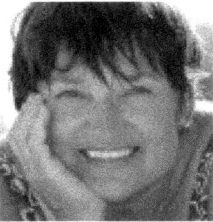

So we are talking about your health – what action are you ready and prepared to take? We have already dealt with the reasons why only you can make the choice about your health and now it is time to ask you some questions and for you to be honest in your appraisal of why these matter, or not, to you.

Honesty: never mind the dictionary definition let's talk about real world honesty where we set aside our fears and possible embarrassment about the things that are personal in our lives.

Things are as they are when you are honest.

X	Question	Why this matters
☐	7.1.1 Are you ready for a change?	In the whirlwind of life it seems there is never enough time to do everything let alone set aside some time for 'you'. A lifestyle that incorporates time for exercise as well as relaxation is a good habit. For many it is not and that is something that many want to change. Is that a change you now contemplate?
☐	7.1.2 What motivates you?	At the beginning of the book there is a list of life's situations that are catalyst to a change of lifestyle to incorporate exercise. Understanding your motivation and desires is important and talks to your attitudes and beliefs. To offer an example, why are some people dedicated to recycling while others don't bother. It is about attitudes and beliefs that lead you to follow a course of action because you regard it as important. Think about this in the context of your health and wellbeing.
☐	7.1.3 Are you a single person?	Most gyms cater for a broad category of memberships and they will allocate the gym's resources accordingly. If you prefer an adult environment then ask to see the gym's rules concerning children on the premises. If you swim check to see what times are allocated to adult only swimming sessions? Are they convenient times for you?
☐	7.1.4 Do you want to make it a joint activity?	Many couples join the same gym and couples usually benefit from a saving on membership - so ask what deals there are for couples. When choosing a gym make certain that it meets both of your requirements. It might be a good idea to visit the gym separately first and then compare your observations. The comments made for a single person in 6.1.3 may also apply.

☒	Question	Why this matters
☐	7.1.5 If you are in a relationship what is your partner's attitude to exercise?	Not everyone feels the same about exercise and this could lead to resentment; you are spending money on a gym membership how does that benefit me? Try to involve your partner but if despite your best efforts this fails then explain your own motivations. You never know as your health and fitness improves they may like the changes (this is often reported) and in turn change their attitude to exercise?
☐	7.1.6 Do you make it a family activity?	Check what facilities are available for children in different age groups. Do they have a crèche? What is the capacity of the crèche? Pick a class taking place in the next week that you would want to attend and check availability of the crèche at that time – they are often busy. How many children activities are there and on what days of the week and times are they timetabled? Do they offer swimming instruction? Are there any other clubs available for children, e.g. a swimming club? The gym is usually off limits for children aged under 16 so check what is available for your teenage children.
☐	7.1.7 Do you play sport or want to take up a sport?	Talk to your fitness instructor about your participation in sports so they can build that into your exercise programme and advise classes that would be suitable. Does the gym have appropriate facilities for your sport(s)?
☐	7.1.8 Are you hoping to meet people and make new friends?	Ask if the gym has a social calendar and 'clubs' within the club. Ask what types of social events they offer, the frequency and the cost (if any) to participate. Ask if 'clubs' exist for swimming, squash, golf, sub-aqua or other activities. Participating in classes advertised in the club's timetable is also a great way to meet people.

☒	Question	Why this matters
☐	7.1.9 Is there a good time to join a gym?	Anytime. The new year (early January) is always a busy time and gyms run promotions to attract the 'new year crowd' and this is one of the busiest times for gyms and they will be at full stretch. The summer is quieter during the vacation months when the weather entices us outdoors. You are about to make a commitment to your health and fitness so anytime is the right time.
☐	7.1.10 Do you have any injuries?	Who hasn't suffered an injury at some time? Exercise can help you recover from injuries. For example, if you have attended a physiotherapist they will treat you and usually advise exercises for you to perform in your own time to aid your recovery. If you have past, recurring or an existing injury then be candid with your fitness instructor. Your health and safety is their highest concern.
☐	7.1.11 Do you suffer from high blood pressure (BP) also known as hypertension?	Many people now routinely monitor their BP at home but you may not so you will not know if you have hypertension. A fitness instructor may test your BP. If your BP is out of a prescribed range, usually $160/100$[9] over two readings, then your fitness instructor may refer you back to your doctor as a precaution before you commence exercise. Blood pressure is a complex subject and your doctor is the best person to provide advice. It is worth noting that one of the factors that increase the risk of hypertension is a lack of exercise.

[9] Around 1 in 4 people have high blood pressure (BP) which is classed as readings consistently above 140/90. A single BP reading is not truly indicative of your BP. If you self-test your BP the recommendation is to take 2 readings day and night over 7 days (28 readings), discard the first day's readings and average the 24 remaining readings. Check out the NHS web site at *www.nhs.uk* for more information.

☒	Question	Why this matters
☐	7.1.12 Are you currently taking any prescribed medication?	Before commencing any exercise you will meet with a fitness instructor who may ask you to complete a PARQ (Pre Activity Readiness Questionnaire). It may ask you if you are currently taking any prescribed medicine. If you indicate that you are then depending on the medication you may be presented with a letter to pass to your doctor to obtain their consent before commencing exercise under the supervision of a fitness instructor.
☐	7.1.13 Do you smoke or been a smoker in the past?	If you smoke, present or past, inform your fitness instructor and they will take this into account when suggesting an exercise programme.
☐	7.1.14 Do you have the right clothing?	Whatever you wear must be comfortable and not restrict movement. When you exercise you will expend energy, get hot and perspire and the clothing that you wear can make a big difference to your comfort and endurance. Two important items of clothing are socks and upper body wear. Buy quality socks, the best that you can afford, as you will need to wash them after each use and they get a lot of wear and tear. Do not wear cotton T-shirts as they get damp with perspiration and then rub the skin. Do buy shirts that are designed to wick away moisture and they wash and dry much more easily than a cotton shirt.

☒	Question	Why this matters
☐	7.1.15 Do you have the right footwear?	Many people don't realise there are big differences in the way sports shoes support your feet. Back, knee and hip pain, Achilles tendonitis, shin splints (leg pain), traumatised toes and painful blisters are some of the conditions arising from wearing ill-fitting or inappropriate footwear. Your footwear is the most important piece of fitness equipment you will buy and wearing the correct footwear can prevent injuries. This is important so there is a section dedicated to choosing footwear in the Appendix.
☐	7.1.16 Do you have a foot care regime?	Because your feet are down there at the end of the body they get far less attention than face or hands and yet they are essential for mobility. If your feet are not in good health and repair then exercise may be uncomfortable or even painful. For advice on care of your feet, refer to the Appendix.
☐	7.1.17 What is your employer's policy regarding encouraging employees to exercise?	Employers know very well the cost of absentee employees through sickness and many are now pro-active in encouraging employees to exercise. Some offer facilities on-site or gym membership within a benefits package. If these don't apply, ask your HR department to consider these options. Involve HR in canvassing employees to determine interest in gym membership and approach gyms about a corporate membership package. Having your gym close to work makes it convenient to exercise before work, during a lunch break or after work.
☐	7.1.18 Are you a key worker?	If you are in a key worker occupation then inform the gym as they may have a membership category for key workers. Be prepared to show evidence that you are a key worker.

☒	Question	Why this matters
☐	7.1.19 Do you qualify for a concession?	It is worth checking so make enquires with your local council leisure department and explain your circumstances. Councils may not offer the same concessions, here is a list of entitlements that might be available based on your circumstances: receiving Job Seekers Allowance, Disability Living Allowance, Attendance Allowance, Pension Credit, Income Support, Working Tax Credit, Full Time Student, Student Nurse, and Full Time Registered Carer. This is not an exhaustive list.

Questions for me

Chapter

8

Questions for them

There are two sides to every Question.

***Protagoras, from Diogenes Laertius, Lives of Eminent Philosophers
(Greek philosopher, 485 BC - 421 BC)***

WHY join a gym when you can buy a celebrity exercise DVD or start running the streets. You have choices so exercise them – go and see what is on offer from gyms they are more than 'gyms'.

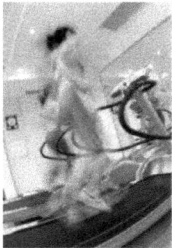

In just about every pursuit in life we need support and that is no different when it comes to our personal health and fitness. The concept of health is easy to understand being the opposite of how we feel when we have a temporary bout of sickness or longer period of ill health. So how should we think about fitness?

This is much harder as for some people having the ability to climb a flight of stairs without puffing and blowing might be a benchmark for fitness and for others that they can ride a bicycle non-stop for 20 miles and complete that in 60 minutes or less.

Gyms attract everyone from those renewing their commitment to an active lifestyle incorporating exercise to competitive sports people. For many people it becomes a social hub where they make friends united in their shared interest in a healthy lifestyle. This variety makes gyms a much more interesting place to exercise than in front of the television watching a repetitive exercise DVD or pounding the streets alone.

☒	Question	Why this matters
☐	8.1.1 Do they offer a trial?	Check the conditions under which you are joining a gym as many commit you to an initial 12-month term. Ask for a trail period prior to joining. If you are not ready to make a commitment look for a gym that offers pay as you go entrance but be aware that may not compare as favourably with the terms of a membership so ask for a comparison if they offer this choice.
☐	8.1.2 What are the Terms and Conditions (T&Cs) of membership?	Read these carefully they are often quite extensive and you should understand what commitment you are entering into – this is a contract. The outline terms will be explained verbally but you must read the T&Cs before signing. The Office of Fair Trading provides a 'Guide to health club membership terms', see Appendix.
☐	8.1.3 What happens if something changes in your life and you need to cancel your membership?	Things can happen that would make it difficult for you to continue to use the gym, for example: a debilitating illness, surgery, relocation by your employer, unexpected financial hardship or moved away making it impractical to get to the gym. Ask about the conditions to release you from your membership if these things were to happen to you and what proof the gym may ask for before agreeing to a release.
☐	8.1.4 Can you suspend your membership? If so what are the conditions for suspension?	You may be temporarily relocated by your employer making it impractical for you to attend the gym (see 7.1.10). Other situations might arise where you need to suspend your membership. However, don't expect a gym to suspend your membership when you go abroad for a holiday.

☒	Question	Why this matters
☐	8.1.5 Is there a joining fee?	Ask why they charge a joining fee. Many gyms ask for a joining fee and it is up to you to consider if you think it is reasonable. It may include some things of value to you like guest passes, a water bottle and towel (but you may have these already). During the year, you may find that the joining fee is reduced or waived according to a gym's need to recruit new members. If you see this advertised then take advantage of it or keep the advert and use it to negotiate with later.
☐	8.1.6 What is NOT included in the membership?	It is worth checking this as the membership may not be all-inclusive, it is sometimes the case that certain activities and classes offered by a gym have a cost. Look at the timetable to check if this might apply to you and factor that into your all up membership fees.
☐	8.1.7 Do they offer a discount if you pay a year in advance?	This could save you money over the year but it may not be refundable (see 7.1.3 before). For some people it is a way to lock in their commitment to attend the gym and get a habit– I've paid for it so I will use it.
☐	8.1.8 How does the gym reward member loyalty?	Gyms want their members to renew their membership so ask how they reward loyalty.
☐	8.1.9 Does the gym have any reciprocal deals?	Many gyms have arrangements with other local businesses such as restaurants and sports shops that offer its members discounts that could save you money that when offset reduces the actual cost to you of your membership. Ask what arrangements they have and how long they have been established.

☒	Question	Why this matters
☐	8.1.10 Is the gym part of a network of gyms?	If you are visiting another part of the country or even outside the country on vacation or business what access do you have to other gyms in the network. If you visit another gym is payment required and, if so, how much? Can you take guests? How much will your guests pay? Do you have to pre-arrange your visit or can you just turn up? What evidence will the gym you are visiting require?
☐	8.1.11 What is the gym's policy regarding a member's guests?	You may want your family and friends to join you occasionally so check what the arrangements are for your guests and guest prices (this may vary according to the activity). If they simply want to join you for a social drink or a meal, do they have to pay to enter the gym?
☐	8.1.12 Is the gym manager available to meet with you?	The gym manager sets the tone for the gym. Ask what changes and improvements they have made recently and why they were required. Were they at the request of members? What changes and improvements are foreseen in the next 12 – 24 months? If you feel comfortable to then share your motivation for using a gym and consider how they reply.
☐	8.1.13 What changes were there between the current class timetable and the previous class timetable?	A class timetable will typically be refreshed every 3 to 4 months and by comparing the current and previous timetables, you will be able to see what changes have occurred. Has the number of classes increased or decreased? Have any new classes been added? Is the number of classes that you have to pay to attend static, decreasing or increasing in number?

☒	Question	Why this matters
☐	8.1.14 How do I book my attendance at a class?	Check how many ways you can book as you do not want to be solely dependent on having to make a telephone call as reception desks at gyms are busy. Can you book online? How far in advance can you book a class? Does the gym operate a penalty system for no shows? If you really want to participate in some classes then before you sign up as a member ask to book some dates/times that would suit you as a way to check availability. This is far more revealing than asking how busy the classes are.
☐	8.1.15 Are beginner classes timetabled?	When you start out you may not be ready to join classes intended for intermediate and advanced users that have a level of fitness and familiarity with a class that develops over time. Learning to perform exercise correctly is important and beginner classes spend more time on instruction. As you become proficient you may want to increase the intensity of your exercise and move up to intermediate and advanced classes that assume proficiency. Check to see what beginner classes are running for those classes that interest you and when they start. Don't be put off if beginner classes are not timetabled as it is usual that instructors ask before starting a class who is new to the class and keep a watchful eye. The first time is the first time for everybody!

☒	Question	Why this matters
☐	8.1.16 Asides from the class timetable what other activities are available?	Some gyms now offer specialist training run over a period of weeks for those participating in sports such as tennis, golf, running, skiing and cycling. This may appeal to you, provide variety and introduce you to other people that you share a sporting interest with. Ask what other activities are available and if there is a cost to participate.
☐	8.1.17 Does the gym have a social programme of events?	Just as you like to exercise sometimes you want to relax and a social event is a great way to meet people that you share a common interest with – health and fitness. It is much easier to make friends when you share a common interest and that might be important to you.
☐	8.1.18 Will you receive a health check and/or fitness assessment?	All gyms operate programmes for the induction of new members but they are not all the same. During your initial 4 weeks, you will need lots of supervision as you will have many questions and need refreshes on how to perform some exercises so check what supervision you will receive. Ask what on-going help you will receive as your level of fitness increases you will require changes to your personalised exercise programme so that you continue to make progress toward your goals. Are there any costs associated with the fitness team reviewing your personalised programme?
☐	8.1.19 Is a personal trainer available?	You might prefer to have 1 on 1 instruction with a personal trainer so ask who is qualified on staff as a personal trainer and the cost. Many people report rapid results from working out with a personal trainer to supervise and motivate you during exercise. If you want fast results then consider the option of a personal trainer.

☒	Question	Why this matters
☐	8.1.20 Are the changing rooms temperature controlled?	Trying to get dry after a workout and a shower can be hard if the changing rooms are hot with high humidity. Do the changing rooms feel cool or hot and damp? Is the floor in the changing area dry or wet?
☐	8.1.21 Are lockers provided?	The answer is almost certainly yes but it is worthwhile to check a number of things. Are they clean inside? Can you hang your clothes or do you have to roll them up to fit in the locker? Are there lockers available when you visit? How is the locker operated, by coin return or padlock?
☐	8.1.22 Is soap and shampoo provided in the shower room?	Not essential but nice to have as it saves you having to buy and carry these products with you.
☐	8.1.23 Can you hire a towel?	It might happen that you forget your towel so it would be convenient to hire a clean towel. If towels are available what is the price to hire a towel?
☐	8.1.24 Is there a spin dryer in the changing rooms?	If you have been swimming then you will want to wash your costume in fresh water and spin-dry it. There is nothing worse than carrying soggy wet costumes in a bag that quickly develop an odour. Some gyms provide a plastic bag for wet items but this is not a substitute for being able to spin-dry your items.
☐	8.1.25 Are hair dryers provided?	If they are and they should be; are they free or do you pay to use?
☒	8.1.26 Is there chilled water dispensed from a water fountain in the gym and changing rooms?	You will receive an explanation about the importance of hydration during exercise so it is essential that a fountain is available to drink from or to fill your water bottle. It is not convenient to have to bring water from home and chilled water is more refreshing.

☒	Question	Why this matters
☐	8.1.27 Is a cleaning rota clearly displayed?	Exercise equipment is used by many people and needs to be routinely cleaned for hygiene. Similarly, changing rooms get messy very quickly if they are not routinely cleaned and tidied.
☐	8.1.28 What catering is available?	Does the gym offer food and beverages or just beverages? Is the menu varied and suit your dietary needs? Is it reasonably priced? What are the opening times? For example, can you grab breakfast after a morning workout before heading off to work?
☐	8.1.29 Is parking free for members? Are there any exceptions to free parking? Is access to parking restricted to members/users of the gym?	If you intend to travel by car, you will want to know that you can park easily. Is access to parking restricted by a barrier? Is the barrier working? Does the car park have lighting as that will be important on dark winter evenings? Does the car park have CCTV? Is the car park owned and operated by the gym? You want to know if the gym has control over access and terms for parking.
☐	8.1.30 Does the gym comply with the FIA Code of Practice?	The Fitness Industry Association (FIA) Code of Practice is designed to ensure that health and fitness operators maintain a basic level of practice to ensure the safety and wellbeing of their customers. Please note that the FIA is a membership organisation so not all gym operators will subscribe to the FIA.

Chapter

9

Other People

To acquire knowledge, one must study; but to acquire wisdom, one must observe.

Marilyn vos Savant (author, lecturer, playwright and listed in Guinness Book of Records under "Highest IQ", 1946 –)

HOW many times have you recounted a story and referred to something about someone else? When that someone has achieved something that you admire how does that make you feel?

Behind your admiration you perhaps wonder what their purpose was, their motivation and sometimes whisper; I could do that if I really wanted to.

Other people sometimes do things that awaken you to possibilities and yet to turn possibilities into reality requires something to happen and that something is - commitment.

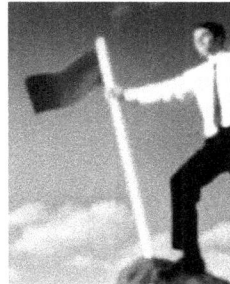

People commit themselves all the time; to study, to work, to care for someone who is sick, to raise children, to volunteer, to a relationship, to a pet and the list goes on. What are your life commitments? Do they include any commitments to your health?

Mostly we do not consciously think about a commitment to our health as we have the expectation that our body will serve us and if it gets sick then we consult a doctor. With a National Health Service that is free at the point of delivery we have a safety net for all our health needs.

In some way, this safety net reduces our concerns about health matters and can diminish the personal responsibility we have for our health and that is plain stupid when you think about it – who else can make the commitment to your health other than you?

If it helps at this point think about someone that has made a commitment and earned your admiration as a result. It has a feel-good factor doesn't it?

Sometimes you might be other people. In an article published in the Financial Times September 3, 2009 under the Business Life section, the reporter responded to the following reader question: Should I employ someone who is fat and spotty? So it would appear that our appearance is something that can be profound in ways that it might impact our life even though that may never occur to us. Now this enlightened reporter gave their verdict that was non-judgmental about a person's appearance and focused on their experience and abilities. I suggest, unlike many people given the question, they were both enlightened and in writing for a national newspaper considerate of political correctness on this subject.

Studies have produced evidence that there is discrimination against overweight people. Search on Google for 'attitudes obesity'. These studies have originated as a result of the growth of obesity in society and the need to understand the implications. Whatever your feelings about this labelling of people, and you may be incensed, this is real world reporting on life.

And so it seems the decisions you make affect the decisions others make about you. That may or may not matter to you?

Here are true stories of some of my clients.

It's all about you

Two attractive middle age women with children both plump joined the gym with the agenda to lose weight and tone up. This was a good scenario as they were in a position to support each other as they set about an exercise programme that I had developed for them. They displayed the usual enthusiasm and attention to following their programme for a few weeks and I, and importantly they, were pleased with their progress. Their transformation was under way. After a time one let their attendance slip and then stopped attending all together. The other carried on. Sometime later they were both standing side by side on a station platform and it was striking to see the difference between the two. One looked trim and fit, had more purpose and you could not help but notice her.

Fell well to Do well

A man in his late thirties presented himself overweight with a BMI of 37 and borderline hypertensive. He suffered from stress and had made a decision to improve his health but had never used a gym. He was a carer for his disabled son and in his own words had neglected his own health and wellbeing that had now culminated in physical difficulties coping with his daily chores and his carer responsibilities. I suggested several changes to his lifestyle and agreed with him an exercise programme. He committed himself to his transformation and over time lost weight to achieve a normal BMI of 25. He now has a lifestyle that incorporates regular exercise and he would tell you that health is a journey, not a destination.

Make life happen

A young man presented himself with the ambition to join the police force but he was underweight and my measurements confirmed this. Having confirmed that he did not have an eating disorder I developed a plan to combine an increase in his daily calorie intake together with toning exercises. An unusual occurrence but worth mentioning to highlight how your health can affect your life choices, in this case this young man's ambition to join the police force.

Get your mojo back

A middle aged man who looked fit and healthy came to me for a gym induction and while watching him complete some exercises it occurred to me that at some time this man had been very fit. I questioned him about his interest in exercise and sport and he revealed that he had been a cyclist and competed in the Tour de France. He was no longer competing but without regular exercise felt he had lost his mojo (his words). I found that interesting as this man had made a connection between exercise and how he felt about himself.

Why wait?

Two women presented themselves, one referred by their doctor the other with the agenda to lose weight and tone up. I put them both through an initial assessment to determine a personal exercise programme and found it interesting to observe the commitment shown by each. The woman referred by their doctor had a wakeup call that she had taken seriously and put effort into the exercises that I asked her to perform. The other was much less committed. Perhaps we can become complacent about our health until something happens that delivers a wakeup call. It led me to think; why wait for a wakeup call.

Check up from the neck up

The stories before tell just a small number of life's situations. When you check up on your health, whether that be your own personal assessment or result of a medical examination, then check up from the neck up. What are your attitudes and beliefs that govern your life choices? Do you consider your health is important and think about your choices and actions to promote good health? On the other hand, will you just leave it to chance?

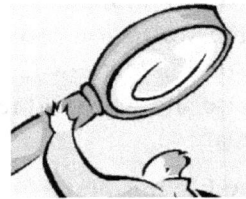

Check down from the neck down

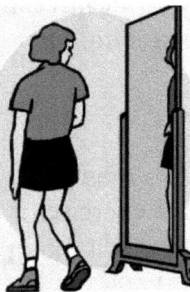

It is a new day; you jump out of bed and stand in front of a full-length mirror. Do you like what you see? Are you energised and ready for this day. Are you looking forward to the exercise you have planned this day, or do you stand there thinking; I really should think about taking some exercise. If you have any nagging doubts go back and read check up from the neck up.

Join in and get started

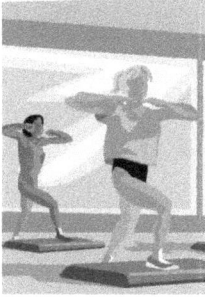

Sometimes we need the inspiration provided by others to make changes in our own life and sometimes we just need help.

One of things I record daily is the fellowship that exists among people that exercise and how they are motivated by others that they workout alongside and that is an intangible yet significant benefit of being a member of a gym.

Other People

Chapter

10

A secret revealed

Advice is what we ask for when we already know the answer but wish we didn't.

Erica Jong (Author, 1942 –)

ONE big learning from the business world could make a big difference in our personal lives. Simply put; our plans are 'easy to say' but generally 'hard to do'.

How do you fix that? I'll share the secret with you that business pay for to get results – setting goals and appropriate measures.

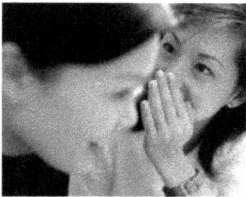

One of the main reasons that people join a gym is to lose weight and the instrument used to measure that is a set of scales. If you weigh yourself every day you will know if you are losing or gaining weight and so the scales become your focus on how you measure your progress toward your goal – to lose weight.

Let me reveal the first secret – this is wrong.

Let me break down what it is you are trying to achieve.

You want to lose weight. This is your goal and your measure is what the scales read when you stand on them. I refer to this as the lag measure and I will explain why in a moment.

In order to lose weight you need to do things that you can influence and is predictable. You can influence what you eat and what exercise you take. In turn, this is how you control your calorie intake (what you eat) and calorie burn (exercise you take).

This is the lead measure and is predictable because when your calorie intake is less than your calorie burn you lose weight.

Here is the second secret. When you measure your weight, the lag measure, all that is telling you is the result about what you ate and what exercise you took - the lead measure. In other words, the scales are 'after the fact'.

It is scientific because weight loss is scientific. You lose weight by measuring (calories) what you eat and what exercise you take. To understand more about this you may find the Food Standards Agency calorie counter instructive, go to *http://www.eatwell.gov.uk.*

The estimated average requirements, a measure of daily calorie intake is: 2550 calories for a man and 1940 calories for a woman[10]. Note: these figures are for a person that has low activity levels (typical of the UK population) and is <u>not</u> overweight. Few people count their calories so you may find the British Nutrition Foundation web site at *http://www.nutrition.org.uk/* has useful information and the intriguing news that you can, eat more and lose weight!

How can you put this in perspective with what you eat and consume in calories.

As noted before, you lose weight when your calorie intake is less than the calories you burn, so how do you know what calories you are burning.

The table adjacent gives some examples.

There are other sources for advice on nutrition and in the Appendix there are directions to NHS web sites that provide information on losing weight and healthy eating.

What a 60kg person burns in 30 minutes:

- running (6mph): 300 calories
- tennis (singles): 240 calories
- swimming (slow crawl): 240 calories
- cycling (12-14mph): 240 calories
- aerobic dancing: 195 calories
- brisk walking (4mph): 150 calories

Source: At least five a week, Department of Health, 2004

---

[10] Source: Department of Health (1991) *Dietary Reference Values for Food Energy and Nutrients in the United Kingdom.* HMSO, London.

You will need to train yourself initially and keep a record of what you eat and what exercise you take. That will soon become habit. You might have this moment; do I really need that chocolate bar? When you hesitate that says you are thinking about changing your habits.

To recap: focus on the lead measure to achieve your goal.

The goal	Lead measure **What I influence and is predictable**	Lag measure **What I will measure and is 'after the fact'**
To lose weight and tone up so I feel fit, healthy and energised	Calories in (what I eat) Calories burned (exercise I take)	My weight My waist and best of all the compliments I receive

A secret revealed

Chapter

11

Final Word

Reading is to the mind what exercise is to the body.

Sir Richard Steele (Writer and Politician, 1672 – 1729)

YOU are the most powerful person in your world when you exercise the power of choice. Others can tell you what they think you should do but only you make it happen.

Sometimes it is so much easier not to make a choice – no decision – therefore I don't fear being right or wrong.

The truth is; you do not get through life by not making decisions and when it comes to your health, you get to make the decisions. Do not fall into the trap of; I'll get to that tomorrow.

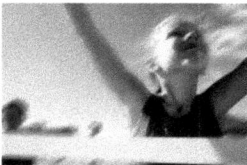

So, think ahead one year from now and imagine some things about your life that you hope will come true. What things come to mind? Do those things in any way depend on you having good health?

Most likely, they do and just as you need good health to support your hopes for the future, so you need good health today.

Appendix - Example PARQ

The use of the Physical Activity Readiness Questionnaire (PARQ) is not universal among gyms. Some use an abbreviated form of PARQ with a few questions (examples below) while others incorporate a detailed lifestyle analysis.

A recent development has been the introduction by some gyms of a 'health commitment statement'. This asks you to state any reason why you should not undertake physical activity that puts the onus with you to make any declaration.

Whichever approach is used it is routine for a new member to be offered a 1 on 1 consultation with a fitness instructor where you can discuss any concerns that you may have in confidence.

The PARQ is structured for you to answer YES or NO to the questions. Examples follow:

1. Have you ever received treatment from your doctor or in a hospital for a heart condition?

2. Do you feel pain in your chest when you do physical exercise?

3. In the past month, have you experienced chest pains when you were not engaged in physical activity (i.e. during relaxation)?

4. Do you suffer any loss of balance or spells of dizziness?

5. Do you have a bone or joint problem that might be aggravated by physical exercise?

6. Is your doctor currently prescribing drugs for the treatment of high blood pressure or a heart condition?

7. Do you know of any other reason why you should not engage in physical exercise?

Note: This is not an exhaustive list of questions to be found in a PARQ.

Appendix – choosing footwear for exercise

It is important to match your footwear to your activity. For general gym work and high impact (jumping and running) activities, you need a supportive shoe with a thick, shock-absorbing sole i.e. a traditional training shoe. Here is some general advice from a podiatrist (foot specialist) about selecting footwear:

- Judge the support of a shoe by its stiffness around the back of the shoe –when you attempt to squeeze the sides of the back of the shoe together you should find it virtually impossible. This support will stop your foot from rolling inwards and is needed by the majority of people.

- Make sure that there is a thumb's breadth, or distance of 1cm, between your longest toe (which isn't always your big toe – check) and the end of the shoe, when you're standing up (your foot generally lengthens when you stand, compared with sitting).

- Don't get shoes that are too big, as your foot will move about too much, which can cause blisters and damage to toenails.

- Wear shoes that have an adjustable fastening, so that you can adjust the fit and make the shoe secure. You cannot do this with slip-on shoes.

- Try shoes on with the type of socks you will wear with that shoe, as sock thickness will affect the sizing of the shoe.

- Ensure shoes are wide enough, as well as long enough (see above). Good sports shops will know which manufacturers offer shoes for wide (or narrow) feet.

- The shock absorption in training shoes doesn't last forever, so replace them every 6-12 months (or every 500 miles).

- Be a savvy buyer and choose comfort over fashion.

Appendix – Care for your feet

Everybody should take good care of their feet, whether they use a gym or not. Taking care of your feet need not take up much of your time:

- Wash feet daily, but do not 'soak' them for prolonged periods in water on a regular basis.

- Dry feet thoroughly after washing – particularly between the toes.

- If you tend to get hard skin on the soles, use a metal foot file several times a week on dry skin. The task is easier when the skin is softer after washing.

- Apply a foot cream daily – this will help to slow down the rate at which hard skin develops and keeps the skin in tip-top condition. Use a cream specially made for feet – containing at least 10% urea (known to soften skin). Never apply cream between the toes – it will encourage fungi.

- Cut toenails regularly and to the shape of the end of the toe – which means rounding off the corners slightly. Don't leave big square corners that can dig into the toe itself.

- Treat signs of fungal infection promptly with Lamisil®, which is available from pharmacies. Signs to look out for are white, wet-looking skin with a 'cheesy' smell between the toes, or little blisters and flaking skin elsewhere on the foot, such as in the arch. If in any doubt, see a podiatrist.

- For further advice on foot care, or for treatment of foot problems, including foot or leg pain, you should see a registered podiatrist or chiropodist (these are interchangeable terms for foot specialists, who must be registered with the Health Professions Council).

- See 'Appendix – Online Resources' for links to finding a podiatrist/chiropodist.

Appendix – Online Resources

For Change4Life activities in your local area with particular help and advice for families:

http://www.nhs.uk/change4life

For advice and information about fitness:

http://www.nhs.uk/LiveWell/Fitness

For advice and information about how to lose weight:

http://www.nhs.uk/LiveWell/Loseweight

For advice and information about 5 a day @Live Well' eat healthily:

http://www.nhs.uk/LiveWell/5aday/pages/5adayhome.aspx

For advice and information about how to quit smoking:

http://www.smokefree.nhs.uk

For The Office of Fair Trading 'Guide to health club membership terms':

http://www.oft.gov.uk/shared_oft/consumer_leaflets/general/oft380.pdf

To find a registered podiatrist/chiropodist in your area, go to the Society of Chiropodists and Podiatrists website:

http://www.feetforlife.org

Links for these web sites were current at the time of publication.

Getting Involved

The Smart Questions community

There may be questions that we should have asked but didn't. Or specific questions which may be relevant to your situation, but not everyone in general. Go to the website (*www.smart-questions.com*) for the book and post the questions. You never know, they may make it into the next edition of the book. That is a key part of the Smart Questions Philosophy.

Send us your feedback

We love feedback. We prefer great reviews, but we'll accept anything that helps take the ideas further. We welcome your comments on this book.

We'd prefer email, as it's easy to answer and saves trees. If the ideas worked for you, we'd love to hear your success stories. Maybe we could turn them into 'Talking Heads'-style video or audio interviews on our website, so others can learn from you. That's one of the reasons why we wrote this book. So talk to us.

feedback@Smart-Questions.com

Got a book you need to write?

Maybe you are a domain expert with knowledge locked up inside you. You'd love to share it and there are people out there desperate for your insights. But you don't think you are an author and don't know where to start. Making it easy for you to write a book is part of the Smart Questions philosophy.

Let us know about your book idea, and let's see if we can help you get your name in print.

potentialauthor@Smart-Questions.com

Notes pages

I hope this book has been a source of inspiration.

As a last thought, if you are ready to do so, make some commitments to yourself about things that you will now do and why it is important to you.

Notes pages

www.ingramcontent.com/pod-product-compliance
Lightning Source LLC
Chambersburg PA
CBHW070931270326
41927CB00011B/2814